AF255110

Self-worth

Peter E Levy

Published in Australia by Ingram Spark
Design & editing: Sharon Hurst

Acknowledgments

While doing my extensive research I quoted and spoke with several psychologists and doctors. I've also quoted several unknown persons, whose work was of a generalist nature. My sincere thanks to you all.

In particular:
Leon F. Seltzer, Ph.D.
Russell Grieger
Cheryl Gale
Martin E P Seligman
Dr. David Kenner

I believe we all learn from each other and I'm very appreciative of any input that furthers self-worth.

Peter E Levy

Contents

Introduction 1
Self-acceptance 3
Personal achievements 10
Positive self-talk 14
Healthy relationships 17
Self-care 24
Continuous learning and growth 29
Helping others 34
Gratitude and mindfulness 40
Criticism and rejection 47
Comparison and social media 50
Trauma and abuse 53

Introduction

I am not a medical person. My knowledge base is purely life experience. Now that mortality is peering over my shoulder, issues, such as this one, is of interest to me and a worthwhile use of my time, intellect, ability and energy.

Please note that I have made every effort to get permissions from the authors/psychologists that I have quoted here. Many thanks and my appreciation to those who did respond positively to that request.

Self-worth is a complex concept influenced by various factors. While it is important to note that self-worth should, ideally, come from within, the reality often lies somewhere else. From personal experience, the imprinting from my parents has been a major contributor to my life, but everybody's experience will be different. What I mean here by imprinting is all those values, attitudes, morals, religious and political affiliations and more, that I was heavily exposed to during my young life. I then came to believe they were my own values and as such tended to judge my self-worth against those values, which in fact were not mine, but had been inculcated in me by my parents and other influences. For example, I often felt guilty and unworthy if I chose to play music with my band on a weekend instead of accompanying my parents to religious services.

So many varying factors can contribute to each individual's values and self-worth, and it is likely that the combined effect of all those factors will hold the key to your personal situation.

Imprinting is a given. We are all subjected to it in one form or another. Understanding that can assist in filtering the self-perceptions that we have come to see as *truths* (many of them may in fact be *mistruths*) that have, over time, found a safe haven in our psyche.

Seemingly harmless words and phrases, from people we trust and depend on, can always trigger these *truths*, for want of a better name, so we must be on the lookout and vigilant at all times. Our self-worth and general mental health depend on us getting correct the narrative of where these truths and mistruths have come from, and what they mean to us.

Self-acceptance

For me, self-acceptance is the first step on my journey to self-worth. There is a proliferation of websites on the topic. I have included here certain quotes that appealed to me most.

[1] *Self-acceptance is the act of recognizing, embracing, and valuing oneself for who you are.*

[2] *Self-acceptance is exactly what its name suggests: the state of complete acceptance of oneself. True self-acceptance is embracing who you are, without any qualifications, conditions, or exceptions*

[3] *"You accept that, as a fallible human being, you are less than perfect. You will often perform well, but you will also err at times. You should always and unconditionally accept yourself without judgment"*

[4] *"[Self-acceptance is] an individual's acceptance of all of his/her attributes, positive or negative."*

[5] *Self-acceptance is an essential ingredient when contemplating personal growth and well-being.*

To achieve a healthy understanding of self-acceptance, requires the courage to actually acknowledge all the positive and negative aspects of your own identity without judgement or self-criticism. We are our own worst enemies.

We can also be our own best friends, too.

When you accept yourself, you develop a more positive and compassionate attitude towards yourself. This, in turn, fosters a healthier self-image and greater esteem. It allows you the freedom to be more authentic, genuine and comfortable in your own skin. This, most definitely, leads to self-confidence and improved relationships with the people that matter to you. Impressing others can mostly take you on a journey down a rabbit-hole where there is no differentiating between the real and the unreal. Not a healthy option, in my opinion. Other people's realities are just that, other people's, not yours.

It is very important to recognize your own worth. That is, to understand that your inherent worth as a human being is not dependent on external factors or achievements. You have a value. You deserve acceptance, simply because you exist.

Several interesting quotes on strengths and weaknesses also caught my attention:

[6]*When you embrace your strengths and weaknesses and celebrate your strengths; your accomplishments will be more meaningful to you.*

[7] For a person to be truly happy and live a meaning-ful life, that person must recognize their personal strengths and use these strengths

[8] A strength is not what you are good at, and a weakness is not what you are bad at. A strength is an activity that strengthens you. It draws you in, it makes time fly by while you're doing it, and it makes you feel strong.

Look around: everyone has weaknesses and areas where they too can improve. It's just not all about you. By accepting your own imper-fections, the prospects to strive for personal growth should be more visible. When the re-alization exposes itself that no one is perfect, the opportunities to embrace humanity and humility will appear less threatening and more enhancing.

[9] Negative self-talk can have some pretty damaging impacts. Negative-self talk has been found to "feed" anxiety and depression, cause an increase in stress levels while lowering levels of self-esteem. This can lead to decreased motivation as well as greater feel-ings of helplessness.

[10] One of the challenges in life is most certainly how we address the narratives we construct and empow-er within our own negative self-talk. (Gleaned from the internet, unknown source.)

You must pay attention and immediately react to these self-critical thoughts. A set of responses, that challenge and reframe those narratives into more positive and compassionate statements, is a strong way to go. Remember to treat yourself with kindness and understanding, in the same way that you would do for a close friend. Healing is the objective here and whatever methodology works best for you, then it's the one to adopt.

It all takes practice. Self-compassion is an excellent way to begin this journey. Simply acknowledge and validate each emotion, as you come across it, without judgement. Then use your self-talk to offer yourself comfort and support when the road gets challenging. And it will get challenging at times.

The main purpose of this book is to ignite a fire of questions. Am I doing what I should do to get the best me that I can? This is your journey and no-one else can take this trip in exactly the way in which you can. There is absolutely no point in comparing your voyage through life with anyone else for many reasons. Your path is unique to you alone. Comparisons generally lead to feelings of inadequacy and self-doubt. Things we do not need at this point in time. Or ever.

I remember hearing Clapton play the guitar so effortlessly and brilliantly, thinking, *what's the point in me trying to be that good?* Luckily, after seventeen movie scores and thousands of songs later, my inferior and somewhat unique style has given me much pleasure. If I had listened to the early narrative, it would have been such a shame. In that particular instance, I quickly decided what were my inadequacies and what original talent I possessed, and worked on the positives, ever mindful that a Clapton or Knopfler I would never be. And once I had come to terms with that *truth*, I did what I did, quite happily.

Just like me, your worth is not determined by how you measure up to others. Come to an agreement with yourself and move on.

When you focus on your strengths you can have opportunity to cultivate gratitude that you in fact have those qualities. The positivity is infectious and will assist in how you view yourself, as well as shifting your perspective towards a healthier self-acceptance.

I have always leaned on my best friends when the going got tough, as it invariably did. Professionals are also always on call when required. No shame in therapy and counselling, as they often provide guidance, support, and a load of different perspectives, as you work through the acceptance of yourself.

There are no quick fixes, in my experience, so a degree of patience is required with yourself. Reward little victories along the way and live in the moment. By embracing who you are and accepting yourself unconditionally, you will cultivate a greater sense of fulfillment, happiness, contentment, and well-being in your life.

1 *The quote "Self-acceptance is the act of recognizing, embracing, and valuing oneself for who you are" is a common statement that encapsulates the concept of self-acceptance. It is difficult to attribute this quote to a specific individual as it represents a widely held belief and has been expressed in various forms by many people over time. The idea of self-acceptance is a fundamental concept in psychology and personal development, and different philosophers, psychologists, and self-help authors have discussed and emphasized the importance of self-acceptance throughout history. (Google)

2 (Leon F Seltzer, 2008). Seltzer, L. F. (2008). The path to unconditional self-acceptance. Psychology Today. Retrieved from https://www.psychologytoday.com/us/blog/evolution-the-self/200809/the-path-unconditional-self-acceptance

3 Russell Grieger, 2013 Unconditional self-acceptance: Be impeccable with yourself. Psychology Today. Retrieved from https://www.psychologytoday.com/us/blog/happiness-purpose/201302/unconditional-self-acceptance

4 da Rocha Morgado, F. F., Campana, A. N. N. B., & Fernandes, M. D. C.

G. C. (2014). Development and validation of the self-acceptance scale for persons with early blindness: The SAS-EB. PloS one, 9(9).

5 (Gleaned from unknown sources on the internet) *The quote "Self-acceptance is an essential ingredient when contemplating personal growth and well-being" does not appear to be attributed to a specific individual. It is a sentiment that aligns with various philosophies, psychological theories, and self-help teachings. Many authors, psychologists, and experts in the field of personal development have emphasized the significance of self-acceptance in fostering personal growth and well-being. Therefore, it is challenging to pinpoint a single person who first uttered this exact quote. (Google)

6 The quote "When you embrace your strengths and weaknesses and celebrate your strengths, your accomplishments will be more meaningful to you" does not have a specific individual attributed to it. It is a sentiment that reflects the importance of self-acceptance, recognizing both strengths and weaknesses, and finding value in one's achievements. This idea has been explored by various authors, psychologists, and self-help experts who emphasize the significance of embracing one's unique qualities and using them as a foundation for personal growth and fulfillment. Therefore, it is difficult to attribute this quote to a single originator. (Google)

7 Martin Seligman date unknown.

8 Marcus Buckingham, 29 Jan 2020

9 (Cheryl Gale, 2020)

10 The quote "One of the challenges in life is most certainly how we address the narratives we construct and empower within our own negative self-talk" does not have a specific individual attributed to it. It expresses a common understanding of the importance of recognizing and addressing negative self-talk, which can significantly impact our well-being and personal growth. Many psychologists, therapists, and self-help authors have discussed the detrimental effects of negative self-talk and the need to change our internal narratives for a healthier mindset. Therefore, it is challenging to pinpoint a single person who first articulated this exact quote. (Google)

Personal achievements

Personal achievements are important. No matter what the size or scale, it is vital that when you set a goal for something and then accomplish that goal, celebrating that moment will truly reinforce your sense of competency and worthiness. So, goal-setting is a powerful tool that allows you to go through a process of defining what it is that you want to achieve and then create a roadmap to get the job done.

The first part of that is actually identifying what your priorities in fact are. Then to reflect on the outcomes that matter most to you to determine core values and aspirations that make sense. Setting realistic goals that align with your true desires sets you on a trajectory that should be hard to distract you from. Becoming a neurosurgeon is not a real goal unless you are already in that medical field of study. You will know the difference when you apply a level of logic in such a way so as not to deflate your sense of worth over striving for goals that were never yours to achieve in the first place.

Clearly define your goals by making them specific, measurable, attainable, relevant, and time-bound. This ensures clarity and provides a clear target to work towards. When you know what you are shooting for and believe in the commitment, there is a higher likelihood you will achieve it on the other side.

Here's a tip. Break your major goals into smaller, bite-sized, manageable tasks or milestones. This obviously makes them less overwhelming and also allows you to track your progress, in real time, along the way.

That brings us to creating a timeline. It is not designed to put you under undue pressure, but a timeline for each goal and its corresponding task will give you a sense of urgency and assist you to stay focused and accountable, to yourself. You know why you are doing it in the first place and there is something deep down inside you that wants to complete it as well.

Find and create many sources that will motivate you. Pieces of paper on a fridge, for example. Gentle reminders that you regularly look at will reinforce the rationale behind the goals. Once you can visualize the desired outcome, track the progress, celebrate the milestones, check in with friends and mentors, you are well set to rock'n'roll.

Of course, things don't always go exactly to plan. That's life, I guess. So, it pays to have some flexibility and not be too rigid with yourself. The end justifies the means. It's ok to adjust and adapt as your circumstances dictate. I have always, in the past, re-evaluated where I was at and, when needed, made the adjustments I felt necessary to me, at the time, so that the end goal remained in sight and was believable and achievable.

If you find flying by the seats of your pants doesn't work that well for you, develop an action plan. Everyone is different. What works for me won't necessarily work that well for you. But if you create a step-by-step action plan, outlining the tasks, resources you have on hand, and the strategies required to achieve the goals, you might find it works better that way. It did for me. My plan, on certain projects, served as a clear roadmap that encouraged me to stay on track.

So, it was important, for me, to regularly monitor my progress. I did this, at times, in a journal and in a diary. Sometimes on scraps of paper that meant something to me and not to anyone else. It helped me assess how I was performing on the tasks and then to make improvements when I felt it was warranted. It also gave me opportunities to celebrate the little wins on the way. Celebrations, like that, are important tools in the overall process.

Even though I see myself as a totally positive person, I expected a certain number of challenges. It is the way each of us handle and overcome the obstacles that define who we are and what resilience we can call on. Staying committed and maintaining a positive mindset are key factors. Learning from each setback and pushing forward with that gained knowledge is a true value-add for now and in the future.

I know I'm repeating myself but it is important to reward yourself at every opportunity. Big and small wins need to be celebrated because it reinforces the level of positivity and motivation required to step over that line as a winner. And, isn't that the reason you started all of this?

Goal setting is a dynamic process. You still have to do the work. It's a tool. Just be open to adjusting your strategies to stay aligned with your ever evolving aspirations and circumstances. It's worth it in the end.

Positive self-talk

I have found that by engaging in positive self-talk and really challenging negative self-beliefs, that this alone will improve your overall self-worth. Try replacing your self-criticism with self-compassion and supportive thoughts. Why not?

Positive self-talk is a powerful tool that can not only boost your self-esteem, but also promote resilience and improve your overall well-being. It's a no-brainer! Some people who accept this in theory, still find they are unwilling to do it. It takes a level of courage and persistence to consciously replace the negative thoughts and words with positive and empowering affirmations. Don't know any? Well, ok, here are a couple to get you started.

I am capable of achieving great things!

I believe in myself and my abilities!

I am worthy of love, happiness, and success!

I am resilient and can overcome any challenge!

I embrace my uniqueness and value my individuality!

I am grateful for the opportunities that come my way!

I deserve to be treated with kindness and respect!

I am in control of my thoughts and my emotions!

I am constantly growing and learning!

I trust myself to make the best decisions for my life!

I have the power to create positive change in, not only my life, but the world!

I am deserving of self-care and self-compassion!

I am confident in expressing my thoughts, ideas and feelings!

I have accomplished many things, and I am proud of myself!

I am surrounded by love and support from those who truly care for me!

There might be some affirmations in that list that don't suit you, just as you might have others to add to it. It's your list . . . manage it well!

Remember, positive self-talk is a habit that requires practice and consistency. By consciously choosing positive affirmations and repeating them regularly, you can gradually rewire your thinking patterns and cultivate a healthier more positive and self-affirming mindset.

Tools, even great tools, don't complete any task. You have to be the master of the tools and actually use them to perform the tasks. I suggest using these tools because they constantly work for me. Give it a go!

Healthy relationships

When you surround yourself with supportive and caring individuals, who value and respect you, the natural consequence will always be an increased level of positivity and self-worth. It must be stressed that this is a two-way street. Mutual respect, mutual trust, and a healthy communication style where no one is talked at, rather, individuals talk with each other. We all know friends who will spout forth, like the turning on of a tap, and dominate each conversation without truly listening to anyone else except themselves. These people are to be avoided or endured in limited doses. Your relationships should ideally include supportive talk and then action, as well as shared values on a multitude of core topics. Well-being and happiness of everyone involved is the primary outcome. Anything less, is copping out on the basic healthy relationship criteria, and could be detrimental to you as well as a waste of time. As one friend succinctly put it, do the test, *is it a gain or a drain?*

Open and honest communication is crucial for building a healthy relationship. It involves active listening, the freedom of expressing thoughts and feelings without judgment or blame, and, importantly, addressing conflicts or issues in a constructive manner. These things seem like no-brainers and easy to achieve with the people closest to you, but the exact opposite is generally the case. It takes time and care to achieve success. Try not to bring up past misdemeanors to win a point. It's worth concentrating on present situations to improve them and leave the baggage in the past.

As in any relationship, trust is the foundation stone. Trust develops from one level to the next, depending on situation, over many years, but is essential to a healthy relationship. Time, gives us all an opportunity to be consistently reliable, honest, and always keeping a given promise. The importance of trust can't be minimized. We all need to feel safe and secure within our relationships. It's pretty much a basic requirement.

From trust, comes mutual respect. How long do I have? I could write treatises about what that means to me, personally, and not reach the end of it. Respect is essential to any healthy relationship. This involves valuing each other's opinions, boundaries, and autonomy. It also requires that we accept the differences we may have while supporting each other's individual growth. What works for one partner should be respected as their thing, even though the philosophy may be totally alien to the other partner. We all bring different strengths to the relationship, and it's that total, combined force that allows each of us to thrive, albeit by different methodologies. That can be hard at times, I know all too well. My philosophy of food intake clashes heavily with my partner's philosophy of less junk equals a better diet. I respect her opinion and it's still a debate as to whether she respects mine. But, it's a healthy debate. That can only come from mutual respect.

In our household, we have a definitive policy of shared decision-making, so that the positive and negative standout points can be put on the table and considered. I would consider my role in that, historically, to be a bit gung-ho, while my partner tends to be always looking for each and every negative aspect. This works very well for us as we are literally forced into considering the other's needs, opinions, and desires, in order to find suitable compromises that benefit both of us. A lot of the time, things come up that we both had initially not even thought of.

This makes good sense to me, as the outcome generally benefits us both in the longer term. Looking at the bigger picture, while entangled in a smaller issue, can be quite difficult to do mid-stream. But definitely worthwhile. Losing some battles and winning the war sees the end justify the means. It's hard to lose or walk away from some battles; it takes working at it.

That means, providing emotional support during the touchy moments. And every relationship has these. My greatest asset, I believe, is that I do offer understanding, empathy, and comfort during those challenging moments. My partner is not too far behind me on that front either. Being there for each other strengthens the bonds we have been cementing since we got together. It is also a lot easier to navigate life's ups and downs with an emotionally supportive partner. I rely on her heavily.

I know that both my partner and I realize that our relationship is not perfect. We used to get trapped by the comparisons of our friends, who, incidentally, we really only saw the best-of - most of the time. While there are undue and totally unnecessary pressures to strive for perfection within a relationship, don't for a minute think that this will suddenly happen instantly. It really is an unreal expectation.

When you embrace the imperfections instead, it opens the door to expose your vulnerability to the other partner, and this is a healthy thing. It's called being authentic. It also has the capacity to form a much deeper connection than you would have thought possible. Acceptance strengthens bonds and teaches us how to grow within the relationship. Compassion, understanding and commitment are the ready-made tools always at our disposal that can help to work through most dramas. So don't despair.

Any two people in a relationship are not totally the same. There are times when all it takes to re-ignite passions is to allow our partners a bit of independence and personal space. It is because we are individual creatures, that it is vital that we maintain separate interests, separate friends, while still sharing quality time and quality activities together. I know there are some friends of my partner who I don't wish to associate with, and I calmly tell her exactly that. In her ambitious zealousness to change my mind on those people, she sometimes opens the door for conflict. On the other side to that, she has the same emotional reaction to some of my friends and family members. After a process of true listening and when the situation still hasn't altered, it's ok. It doesn't matter what the rationale or back-story to any of these conflicts is. What does matter, is that we both can accept that we each have the right to feel that way. That's another important form of respect.

Although not a pre-requisite, it is a lot easier when both partners are on the same page about major issues. For example, If I was a Trump supporter and she wasn't, that would be a deal-breaker. Luckily, we share similar values on that front. We also share the same religious values too. None! The element of cultism that exists in all religions is one we stay clear of, while still maintaining a healthy spirituality. We just don't require the added rituals that are required to participate in any structured religion. They are major issues. I don't feel we could have survived if we were in opposing camps on just those two issues. There are plenty more, and friends have come and gone, through our choices, directly as a result of it too. It is alright to have differing opinions, but it is not alright to continually make either of us feel uncomfortable or guilty about them. We follow the science. Show me the facts. Where is the source for your belief? And the rest sorts itself out logically. We both have strong personal attachments to Christian and Jewish clergy, who we both respect and accept. That doesn't mean we agree with the philosophy or rituals of those religions. Very clearly, we don't.

What is important to us, is that we kiss each morning and re-avow ourselves to each other. We tell each other that we love the other and exhibit kindness, gratitude and physical affection no matter where we are. It's a process of continuing the nurturing within a safe and healthy environment. And, while I can share our experiences, everyone else's relationship is personal and unique. What works for us may not work for you. I repeat it, only because it really needs repeating and reinforcing, and, as said before, is an essential ingredient in the journey towards self-worth.

Self-care

You may have had the experience while traveling on a plane, when the lights flash and the air-bags drop down. Or, without such a dramatic scenario, then you may remember the flight attendant indicating the air-bags and the clear, calm voice over the intercom instructing us to place the masks on ourselves first before attempting to do so for any small child in our care.

It may have sounded weird at first, but the solid philosophy behind the command indicates the principle behind self-care. We are of no use to anyone, let alone ourselves, if we constantly put the needs of others above our own. Make sure you prioritize self-care activities, such as exercising, eating well, getting enough sleep, and engaging in hobbies and pursuits that bring joy, as all these things contribute to a sense of self-worth.

Self-care refers to the practice of taking care of your own physical, mental and emotional well-being. It involves engaging in activities and behaviors that promote personal health and happiness. So essential for maintaining a balanced and fulfilling life, especially in today's fast-paced and stressful world.

While supposedly sleeping, when I have a new song lyric floating in my brain, I tend to get out of bed and write it down. It helps me on one level, that I don't forget the line or two, but it also is terrible for my sleep patterns. Even though I justify it to myself, by writing a new song, the damage to my health is undeniable. It was the same when playing gigs at all hours of the early morning. Being on such a high is totally detrimental to my sleep. While in those experiences, I tended to disregard all the warning signs, but I now identify them as vitally important. My recommendation is not to follow, if you can, what I did on those issues.

My daily regime consists of a healthy breakfast followed by regular and vigorous exercise. As an ex-sportsman, exercise was a given. So, I trained hard and ate hard. I was lucky in that regard. I also maintained a practice of medical check-ups just to be sure, to be sure.

By eating hard, I am talking about nachos at every possible occasion, fish'n'chips whenever I was tempted, KFC wicked wings, and plenty more of the foods I actively limit, these days.

My emotional self-care was often expressed in my songs and novels, and I'm told that I'm quite a weeper when it comes to sad movies. I have a couple of very close friends who encourage me to chat about personal issues, and I always come away from such discussions a lot happier and healthier.

Mentally, I do regular sudoku puzzles and am always involved with learning a language on Duolingo. My latest is Chinese. Don't ask me what I remember (ha). It's the thing of doing it every day that keeps my brain (hopefully) healthy, and I believe it delays dementia. Nothing to lose on that front if I'm wrong about it, either.

Socially, my wife and I have many friends and the pleasure of many reciprocal dinners. Conversation around the meal table can flow from superficial to deep and meaningful – and that's ok. We also attend university lectures when we can as well as our local council functions. Our close friends get the true one-on-one interactions that extend beyond dinner parties into something I treasure greatly. I know there are three people I could ring, any time of the day or night, if I needed to. They know they can do the same to me as well. That's what true friends bring to the table. Think about how many you could call on.

For my spiritual self-care, I have tended to overlook all of the regular religions as I didn't want to get caught up in any cult beliefs or the baggage that is expected of you when you immerse in them. I'm sure that a lot of people will get exactly what they are looking for in traditional religion-based spiritual caring, but it's not for me, and luckily, not for my wife either. I have tended to randomly choose two of the eight rules associated to Bushido. When I do this, I endeavour to think about the chosen rules whenever I have a decision to make. This current month my Bushido choices have been, self-control and mercy. This works for me.

What is also important for self-care is saying no to things. I know I can't be everything to everyone and it's even pointless and futile to even attempt it. Having said all that, it was always my agenda to be liked by everyone. Not now! I set boundaries on almost everything I do these days. I'm still a workaholic but I've culled friendships that were too one-sided, and pretty much anything I consider to be a drain on my dwindling resources. It's right across the board. Either I gain from you and you gain from me or you simply drain me. If you drain me, I'll soon be out of there. Life is too short to waste it. We all have to protect ourselves in the clinches, and this is one strategy I employ to do just that.

At the end of the day, as my daughter often says, we all need to have respite time by way of relaxing activities. That will mean different things to different people. I love long walks, enjoy my sudoku, enjoy writing, singing and creating. Sometimes, it's a fine line between what is a hobby and what is a driven passion. But, that's just me. Find your own ways of expressing enjoyment throughout your leisure time. It is very rewarding to your overall health and vital to your self-care. I know that I come out of those times more energized and totally better equipped to handle life's challenges. Whatever they might be.

Continuous learning and growth

Continuous learning and growth are crucial aspects that affect all areas of your self-worth. Be they keeping abreast of some of the advances in your own area of expertise or just being curious about the changing world we live in; it is all a further benefit. I find that by being open to new ideas and perspectives adds a spark. Every spark is important. Some new knowledge is relevant. Not all. But it does give you and me an opportunity to enhance skills we already possess.

Continuous learning also contributes significantly to personal growth by expanding your understanding of the world. It fosters critical thinking as well as enhancing problem-solving abilities. And, don't we need them, at the moment? This, of course, leads to an increase in self-confidence, a much broader perspective, and the ability to adapt to new situations and challenges, better. This is an ever-changing world in which we find ourselves, and there is nothing we can do to change that. Better to be equipped, properly, I say.

Continuous learning can take on many forms, quite apart from formal education. We should be open to different, diverse learning methodologies as we guide ourselves through the quagmire. Essentially, by allowing new ideas and concepts to filter slowly into the hallowed turf of our "established" ones, surprising things will occur. How? you might ask. Informal reading, online courses, attending workshops and seminars, participating in webinars, engaging in hands-on experiences, or seeking mentorship from experts. You could also offer yourself as a mentor to others, like my wife and I are doing, in areas that we are strong in. If you think about it, I'm sure the possibilities for many of these activities, and many more, will present themselves, and now you might identify them and be more proactive. I can only hope so, for your well-being.

Adopting a growth mindset is crucial for continuous learning and growth. It involves believing in the capacity for improvement. It also involves embracing challenges, setbacks, and failures as positive opportunities. I tend to learn little when gliding from success to success.

True learning and understanding can only come from failures. When you plant a seeding and it grows happily into a luscious bloom, you take it for granted and enjoy the fruits of your labor, maybe without a second thought. However, if your seedling dies, you may reflect upon what caused it. Hence you hopefully become a better gardener. This analogy can be taken into your personal growth journey. When you experience failure, it may do you a favor, if you can reflect deeply enough on your own contribution to that failure, and learn from the experience.

Don't be too hard on yourself. Set achievable goals and continue to push the boundaries. In that way you will, eventually, reach an enlightenment on the field of your enquiry and search. With continuous learning, as in many other things, it is the journey, not the destination that is important and relevant to your progress.

During this process, I would recommend constant reflection on your experiences so that you can identify areas where you excel as well as areas that require improvement. A simple adjustment in strategy can assist you in making more informed decisions moving forward.

You will never know it all. Things change. By interacting with others and networking by sharing information, we can often accelerate the learning process and broaden our perspectives. In this way we can avoid the many pitfalls and one-way streets, as well as understanding the errors. Like-minded people are always interesting to each other. They are on the same quest and share some of the values you may have.

It's all about being adaptable, being open and embracing changes and new ideas. There are many learning opportunities if you are pro-active enough to seek them out. Staying up to date with advancements in your own field of interest makes sense, doesn't it?

Looking after the physical side of your body is just as important as maintaining a healthy mindset. It is somewhat crucial to create a balance between them, too. Fostering healthy relationships is essential for sustained growth and overall life satisfaction. You are probably in a healthy relationship, but don't get complacent about it. It is a rare gift. Take nothing for granted. Respect and nurture it while you bless your lucky stars that you indeed have it. I know I do. If you are in the midst of an unhealthy relationship, my suggestion would be to try and improve that status as best you can. It may work and is certainly worth a try. If it doesn't work, and you've tried various approaches, consider self-protection options.

Continuous learning is a lifelong commitment to acquiring new knowledge, developing skills, and embracing personal and professional development. Who knows what could result from it? It's definitely worth it and I wish you luck. Yes, there is some luck to it, but winners make their own luck. All you need to do is have the mindset and determination of a winner. Not easy, but achievable. If one person can do it, so can you.

Helping others

Acts of kindness and helping others can enhance self-worth by providing a sense of purpose as well as making a positive impact on the lives of others. It is a wonderful way to make a positive impact on the world, too. The butterfly-effect actually works, even if we can't see it happening. It is constantly occurring. Improving the lives of people around you, in your community or family, has so many benefits, both in the short-term as well as the bigger picture. Sometimes, that bigger picture gets a bit blurred due to it being so overwhelming and beyond the limits of our capabilities. Remember that mighty oak trees started from a single seed. We all can make a difference, both individually and as a joint cooperative.

When you offer your time and skill sets to non-profit organizations, community centers, hospitals and schools, you will receive the respect and thanks from all the other volunteers. There are many ways to contribute. Tutoring, mentoring, organizing events, or just by providing support to those who you consider to be in need.

You may even think about donating money, clothing, food, or other items to charities or local shelters. Many organizations depend on donations to provide the vital resources to individuals and families who have fallen on hard times and the government has simply neglected. I know of several people who only survive from pay cheque to pay cheque. One glitch in their fragile system, like an injury or a sickness, could see them on the streets, just like that. When I drive around our city and some of the suburbs that have many restaurants and cinemas in them, the numbers of homeless people seem to be getting larger. You will not be able to solve every problem like that, but by donating to worthwhile causes and charities that actually assist people in distress, you would have to feel better about yourself. Your self-worth, as a human being, will benefit from these actions as well.

If it is within your capability to organize fund-raising events, or simply to campaign to raise money for a cause you care about, this also is very worthwhile. Your own network of family, friends and work colleagues could also be useful in such ventures to maximize the efforts. So, there is much you could do, if you really wanted to help. I know that I need to do more on that front and am determined to do so in the future.

Closer to home, by supporting local business-es, such as a deli or milk-bar, instead of the large chain supermarkets, it will stimulate the economy where you live. This will have a cause and effect on the positive growth of your own community. So, you might pay an extra dollar for a litre of milk, or a few cents extra for fresh vegetables, but the survival of these enterpris-es is important. Think of it as a convenient way to chat to neighbours, rather than having to park in overcrowded bustling carparks. Look at the advantages and weigh it up against your own economic needs.

We all possess special skills and expertise in something. The trick is finding out early what that gift is for you. Another way of enhancing self-worth is to share those skills with others. Offer free workshops or teach a class or two. I am always on the assist to budding songwriters to let them glean knowledge from what skills I've honed over the years. The truth is, I learn so much from them as well. My skill sets have the tendency to become routine and wooden.

That is so easy to happen, too. A new song can sometimes sound like the last song. Or, I use similar lyrics without noticing it. I try to be mindful that this is happening, but not always. By working on other people's work and honing their skills, I learn a lot. Always learning. My wife and I, over many years, have mentored various people in subtle ways that lead to solid friendships rather than a teacher to student relationship. Mentoring is also a two-way street, and I'm grateful for the opportunity to participate in it. We still do it, whenever we can. The current flow of refugees from Syria and Africa are always happy to learn our cultural ways to fit in, just as I am very interested in their cultures as well.

Six months ago, I saw an animated film about a lost boy and a mole. The mole casually asks the boy what he would like to become when he is older. "Kind," said the boy. That has resonated with me from the minute I heard it. How profound is that? Simple acts of kindness can go a long way. Try offering a listening ear to someone going through a rough time, provide words of encouragement, or just listen, or simply perform an act or two of kindness to brighten up someone's day. People do that for me and I always appreciate it and never take it for granted. And, neither should I. Truly listening is a skill. Some people have a lot of issues with listening as if it poses an opportunity to turn on their tap and hold the floor with a barrage of words. That can be very draining. The old question remains: *Is it a drain or is it a gain?*

On a larger scale, this planet we call Earth has dire needs with disasters around every corner. While you won't have the ability to totally stop some, or all, of them, you can do your bit. There are always clean-up drives to get rid of the plastic. I'm sure you could find like-minded souls to plant trees with and educate people about sustainable practices within your community. You have a voice, so use it. Express your opinions and concerns whenever and wherever you can. Organized rallies and meetings are ideal for this activity but not necessary for it. You elected politicians to work for you, so contact them and become more pro-active on the issues you are genuinely concerned about. In Tasmania, Bob Brown saved the Franklin River, and people got behind some of his initiatives to stop over-logging. Very worthwhile causes in my mind.

I know I've mentioned volunteering before in this book, and I'm sure I've repeated myself several times, but it's because certain issues need reinforcing into our psyche. Natural disasters offer ideal opportunities to volunteer, but you don't need to wait for one. Feeding the poor from caravans in selected areas is always on, so you don't have to look far. Helping the poor is a wonderful way of enhancing your self-worth.

The act of helping others is not only beneficial to those receiving the assistance, but can also bring fulfillment, joy, and a sense of purpose to your own life. Think about it. Start small, find causes that resonate with you, and gradually expand your efforts to make a positive impact on a larger scale. It's called the power of one. It's also great fuel for self-worth.

Gratitude and mindfulness

Practising gratitude and being mindful of the present moment can promote self-acceptance and appreciation for what you have, contributing to increased self-worth. G & M are two powerful practices that can bring numerous benefits to our lives. While they are distinct practices, they complement each other in so many wondrous ways, that they are often practised together. But that doesn't necessarily negate the individual practices; both ways are important.

Gratitude is the practice of recognizing and appreciating the positive aspects of our lives. It involves acknowledging the good things we have, the experiences we already enjoy, and the people who support us. Practising gratitude regularly can cultivate a positive mindset, improve our overall well-being, and enhance our relationships. It helps shift our focus from what may be lacking in our lives to what we already have, fostering a sense of contentment and fulfillment.

Mindfulness, on the other hand, is the practice of intentionally paying attention to the present moment without judgment. Some years ago, my wife and I spent two and a half years studying philosophy at the Royal Academy in the heart of Melbourne. Every Tuesday night for four wonderful hours. One of the key points I gleaned from the experience was what they called *the exercise*, whereby we all had to focus on the present moment, starting with our breathing and extending to things we could feel, see and hear in our immediate surroundings. This theory extended to discussion, and we were encouraged to only discuss topics that we had actually experienced.

"Talk about what you know," the group leader told us. "Don't pass judgment or be too opinionated on those things you have not personally experienced." Often what you think you know has been filtered through the eyes and hearts of someone else. Just like our childhood imprinting, in which much of who we become and our beliefs are shaped by things that have been inherited, so *the exercise* removed preconceptions from the table by disassociating them from our own lives. They weren't ours.

All sorts of discriminations that have been passed down the ages, like antisemitism, fear and hatred of black people, Islamophobia, family feuds, hatred of another's sporting club, hatred of a certain ethnic group etc. These prejudices are simply not ours.

Think of the Middle Ages and even before that, when there was a largely illiterate population fed all sorts of non-truths by organizations, like church pulpits. So, fear, hatred, and prejudice became people's realities when in fact, they really weren't. It was the agendas of other organizations.

The exercise helped me to see past the indoctrinations all around me and try to eliminate them from my overall views and judgments of the world, because they were NOT my experiences.

Take judgment and jealousy out of the narrative. Observe your own thoughts and see where that journey takes you. Mindfulness helps us to become more aware of our own experiences and enables us to respond to them in a non-reactive and compassionate manner. Regular mindfulness practice can reduce stress, increase self-awareness, improve concentration, and enhance our overall mental and emotional well-being.

When combined, gratitude and mindfulness can amplify their individual benefits. By practising mindfulness, we become more aware of the positive aspects of our lives, making it easier to cultivate gratitude. Similarly, cultivating gratitude can deepen our mindfulness practice by providing us with a positive foundation to observe and appreciate the present moment. And isn't that all we really have? The past is long gone and out of reach, the future is an unknown thing and not accessible by we mortals. The present is really all we have access to. It is our world.

I used to write down the things I was grateful for on scraps of paper, and then incorporate them in my songs and novels. In that way, I could reflect on each of the points, no matter how insignificant and small they were, and again express gratitude whenever I read and re-read them. The power of song lyrics is amplified a thousand times when you hear it in your own voice. Your voice is well known to your mind and is an instant portal into the deepest crevices of your psyche. This alone is something I am grateful for too, as not everyone has that talent or ability. The songs themselves are by no means great or even good by the standards of other artists that I respect. But they are mine. My lyrics, my voice, my mind.

Another aspect of *the exercise* was to find pleasure, no matter how small, in things around me, without judgment. As a voracious eater, so I'm told, I now know to limit the amount of tomato sauce I used to splash on everything so that I could savour the actual taste. My mother, on my wedding day, said to my first wife, "A barrel of tomato sauce is really all you'll need to satisfy his hunger. He won't taste anything else." There was of course a lot of humour mixed into the wisdom of it too. My mother was a great cook and I do regret not fully appreciating that at the time. My current wife is also a great cook, and I try very hard to appreciate every morsel. I also express gratitude, very regularly, for the healthiness of the food as well as the delicious flavours.

Healthy eating habits are important and I still have a way to go on that front. I love cornchips, cheese and jalapenos, and used to eat them six or seven times a week. I don't do that anymore, but the thought still lingers. Like a fat cigar after a hearty meal. Where did that come from? Probably the American movies. I

threw out all my cigars and pipes when my wife
and I decided to go cold-turkey on all forms
of smoking. Good decision too. My sport
improved as my lung capacity got back some
of its vibrancy, and I'm sure I was headed for
lung-cancer down the track at the rate I was
abusing my body. Just like coffee. In former
times, working at a recording studio in Perth,
my cup was constantly being filled and refilled.
I was on a constant high.

These days, after much negotiation, I am down
to one cup of black coffee a day. I choose mid-
day so that I have something to look forward
to that won't necessarily affect the little sleep I
get. I'm still a workaholic. This change in my
lifestyle has in turn dramatically improved my
health and my feelings of self-worth

The exercise also encouraged me to do my own
version of meditation and I am constantly
drawn into my own head, much to the annoy-
ance of everyone else. The meditation aspect
of the philosophy course was, funnily, the rod
that broke the camel's back. We were invited
to tithe a portion of our income when we, as a
group, practised meditation. I objected to that
as it smacked too much like the tithing of re-

ligious orders and cults, so decided there and then to take all the good points learned, with gratitude, and do my own thing. Luckily, my wife came to the very same conclusion.

Gratitude and mindfulness are skills that like others, require practice. If you can incorporate them into your daily routine the benefits will far out-weigh anything else. Try it. The reward will be greater happiness and greater well-being, and that in turn will give you a greater self-worth.

The road I travel through life would be totally unnavigable without the support of a loving wife, good friends and professional advice, when I feel I require it. We were never built to master everything and a chat with a close friend about an issue I am facing, that may be similar to what my friend is experiencing, enhances my resilience and of course strengthens my self-worth. And that's what this book is all about, isn't it? I acknowledge and appreciate all the help I have received and still am receiving, along my journey, and why not?

Criticism and rejection

Repeated criticism, rejection, or negative feedback from others can erode self-worth over time. When any of us face constant judgment or feel consistently unaccepted, it can lead to a diminished sense of self-worth. And, it is generally unfair as well as being unhealthy to all concerned. The receiver as much as the deliverer. Criticism and rejection are common aspects of life that can be very challenging to handle, but they do offer opportunities to rise above them and experience growth and self-improvement.

Remember that criticism and rejection are subjective opinions and not definitive judgments on your worth or abilities. Everyone shares differing perspectives, and what one sees as a flaw, another may perceive as a strength. The most valuable diamonds in the world all possess a flaw that makes them unique and special. So why not us?

When criticized or rejected, I tend to self-reflect and evaluate my role in all of that. In a lot of cases I see areas of self-improvement so I view constructive criticism as a useful tool to further my growing and learning. I never let it influence the way I evaluate or validate my self-worth, as my self-worth does not depend on the approval and/or acceptance of others. My self-worth is based on my own intrinsic values and accomplishments, rather than coming from a casual slap-on-the-back comment or throwaway line from someone else.

I do, however, learn a great deal from setbacks and rejections. In the case of my passion for music, there have been plenty of those over the years and they do hurt a bit, that's for sure, but there are always valuable lessons and insights to be gleaned. I've learned that, rather than take those rejections personally, for me it is more important and fulfilling to pursue my own journey, even though it may not follow the trend or be in the mainstream.

Fake it till you make it was my motto and driving force when I first settled in Melbourne. It worked for me. But if my style didn't appeal to the masses, there was little to be gained by crying about it. Just analyze the feedback, identify areas to improve, and then refine your skills accordingly when you next dip your toe into the water. If you are tenacious and totally believe in the approach you are taking, as well as the quality of the product you are submitting, then I say, go for it again. You may not succeed and the formula for success varies all the time, but for your own peace of mind, keep doing it. Remember, it's the journey, not the outcome. Some people never make it in their chosen field and that's just a sad fact of life.

As always, seek advice from the pros as well as your network of family, friends and mentors. They can help put your mindset back to the job at hand. Navigating criticism and rejection is hard. Nothing worth anything comes easily without a price attached. It's resilience and persistence that are important. You can't get that magical call that you will be lining up for the team, if you're no longer in the game. Stay the distance and stay focused. There are no guarantees; there never were any.

Remember, don't take every criticism and rejection as personal. Just see them as obstacles that need to be overcome, challenges that need to be embraced and conquered, motivation tools to keep you in the right direction. All this takes time and patience. There are generally no quick fixes, just stepping stones from experience towards your own personal and professional growth.

Comparison and
social media

Constantly comparing yourself to others, particularly through the lens of social media, may only lead you down a rabbit-hole towards feelings of inadequacy and lower self-worth. Seeing curated and idealized versions of others' lives can sometimes lead you to believe that you don't measure up. But you are looking at a highly orchestrated PR machine at work that may have little to do with reality as we know it. Don't get sucked in by it.

Because social media has become such an integral part of our daily life, shaping how we communicate, gathering information, and interacting with each other, I cannot resist diverging here to examine how I perceive this latest overwhelming phenomenon in our lives.

Sure, I'm as guilty as the next person of using social media to enhance my feelings of self-esteem. I promote my music and novels via platforms like Spotify, Facebook, Twitter, etc . . . no big deal, really. But different social media platforms serve very different purposes.

Facebook was originally just a friend-to-friend platform that has evolved into a multipurpose platform for sharing content, joining groups, and following pages.

Twitter is probably best known for its short-form posts, or tweets, and their focus is more on real-time, as well as information sharing. There are plenty of public conversations going on too and I, at times, add a link to a song of mine just to get more hits.

Instagram is a more visual platform and revolves around sharing photos and videos, with a strong emphasis on aesthetics and lifestyle. If you are an influencer, then there are opportunities to reap real monetary rewards from the fact that you have many hundreds of thousands of followers. Probably more geared to the twenty to thirty-year-olds. Somewhat superficial. Both for the influencers and the influenced, but it is a marketplace.

LinkedIn is probably my favourite as it is business to business in its approach. My experience has been to link up with musos all over the world and for me it has been very successful. Some of my songs are now recorded by artists in the USA as well as other countries, which is a bonus and thrill for me and cannot help but boost my feelings of self-worth.

There seems to be an ever-increasing number of these platforms but I tend to use only four of them. While all can be wonderful tools for self-worth enhancement, with the holy grail of as many thumbs-up likes as you can get, just be aware again that this is not critical to your self-worth, and can sometimes be just an ego trip. And a further warning, don't go down rabbit holes of misinformation, a scourge dominating today's world.

All that said, and having pointed out the positives of social media, don't forget the dark side to this phenomenon: cyberbullying, online harassment, hate speech, and maybe even the absence of likes can lead to mental health issues such as stress, anxiety and depression.

It's easy to get addicted. Getting likes and hits is a fuel for most egos and I'm not immune to it either. When one of my songs is getting half a million hits, my mind and heart can skip a beat. It is what it is. Nobody is perfect, especially me.

Trauma and abuse

Experiencing traumatic events or being in abusive relationships can significantly impact self-worth. Physical, emotional or sexual abuse, as well as neglect, can leave deep emotional scars and make individuals feel unworthy or undeserving of love and respect. It is crucial to seek professional help from therapists, counsellors, psychologists and police departments that deal in trauma if you're able to do so.

I do not represent, nor have been trained, in any of these areas. So, my key advice is for you to seek assistance from people who have been trained in this field. They have the expertise to provide you with the necessary professional support, guidance, and coping strategies tailored to your specific and personal situation. I do of course have a few suggestions of my own.

I would say that it is important to share your experiences with trusted friends, family members, or support groups so that you feel less isolated and alone. By cultivating a healthy lifestyle, like getting a good night's sleep, eating a balanced meal, engaging in hobbies and generally trying to relax through meditation, a clearer way forward should present itself. That way you hopefully avoid rushed and rash decisions that can ultimately put you in further danger.

Obviously, this is a highly fraught area, constantly spotlighted in today's media. Even experts seem unable to solve the burgeoning problems of abuse in our society. But what do I know? I do see education as vital. If you can get some insight into what is happening to you and understand that a healing process does exist, it may empower you. Nothing will be easy, but if you have the knowledge and the will, my advice would be to reach out and do everything possible to change your life for the better. We only have one life – this is not a dress rehearsal.

If you are a victim of domestic violence and you are planning to leave, my suggestion would be, if possible, to squirrel money away, so that when the time is right, you are somewhat prepared, both financially and mentally. It is probably also wise to let professionals, like the police, know what is on your mind and your resolve to change your life.

There will be a lot of blame floating back and forth, as well as denial of the realities of the situation. Sometimes, there might be cultural boundaries you may feel unable to cross, but I suggest it is worth the pain and effort to cross them, to live a better life. We all deserve that. Yes, there will be setbacks along the way and no-one will guarantee any segue that will make the journey easier. Your self-worth depends on what you do, and by not doing anything, I'm sure you will dig a big hole where you could feel useless, incompetent, and have an ever lowering of your self-esteem. So, do something!

Everyone, I'm sure, experiences this type of situation differently, so be patient and gentle with yourself as you work through your difficult situation and hopefully arrive at the healing process.

Constant brutalizing, be it criticism or physical abuse, can become so ingrained that it might seem normal. It isn't, I can assure you. Normal looks and feels very different. Luckily, my wife and I have a good relationship built on solid foundations. It may have taken me a few marriages to reach the understanding of what that meant, but I wanted to go down that path so that a fuller experience of intimacy was available for me to experience. I have not been disappointed at all. I have lost nothing and gained a better life. You can too.

Some people get trapped in their situation through the onset of mental illness, and that is a hard thing to deal with on top of a worsening living environment. So, act now, sooner, rather than later, to try and avoid that happening.

***

It's important to remember that self-worth is a lifelong journey that can be rebuilt, restarted and strengthened as you work towards building a positive self-image. Be kind and resolute to yourself, the first step to achieving a stronger self-worth. One day at a time is what it takes, so long as you have a positive narrative in your head reinforcing every step you take.

Keep telling yourself that you deserve to live better . . . because you indeed do deserve it. Everyone does.

Good luck.